Care-giver's Journ

MW00466085

This Journal Belongs to

Name	
Contact Number	Email
Address	

Care Recipient Info

Name	
Birth Date	Age
Address/ Contact Info	

Emergency Contacts

Name	
Contact Info	
Name	
Contact Info	

Journal Info

Journal Start date	
Journal Number	

"Hope is the only bee that makes honey without flowers."

Robert Green Ingersoll

Designed and created using free resources from: pixabay.com, rawpixel.com, freepik.com, vecteezy.com, unsplash.com

Medical Professionals Contacts

Name	
Info	
Name	
Info	
Name	
Info	
Name	
Info	
Name	
Info	

Chronic Conditions / Allergies

Drugs & Medications

Name	Dosage	Timing

Insurance Details

Provider	
Policy Start Date	Policy End Date
Coverage	
Contact Info	
Website	
Email	

Insurance Details

Provider	
Policy Start Date	Policy End Date
Coverage	
Contact Info	
Website	
Email	

Insurance Details

Provider	
Policy Start Date	Policy End Date
Coverage	
Contact Info	
Website	
Email	

Daily Journal

Date: ....

Caregiver: ....

Sleep	Weight	Blood Pressure	Fluids Intake

Feeling: ....

DRUGS & MEDICATIONS	DOSAGE	TIMING

MEALS	TIME	NOTES

Tasks & Activities

....

....

....

....

Concerns / Notes

....

....

....

....

Daily Journal

Date: ....

Caregiver: ....

Sleep	Weight	Blood Pressure	Fluids Intake

Feeling: ....

DRUGS & MEDICATIONS	DOSAGE	TIMING

MEALS	TIME	NOTES

Tasks & Activities

....

....

....

....

Concerns / Notes

....

....

....

....

Daily Journal

Date: ....

Caregiver: ....

Sleep	Weight	Blood Pressure	Fluids Intake

Feeling: ....

DRUGS & MEDICATIONS	DOSAGE	TIMING

MEALS	TIME	NOTES

Tasks & Activities
....
....
....
....

Concerns / Notes
....
....
....
....

Daily Journal

Date:

Caregiver:

Sleep	Weight	Blood Pressure	Fluids Intake

Feeling:

DRUGS & MEDICATIONS	DOSAGE	TIMING

MEALS	TIME	NOTES

Tasks & Activities

Concerns / Notes

Daily Journal

Date:

Caregiver:

Sleep	Weight	Blood Pressure	Fluids Intake

Feeling:

DRUGS & MEDICATIONS	DOSAGE	TIMING

MEALS	TIME	NOTES

Tasks & Activities

Concerns / Notes

Daily Journal

Date: ....

Caregiver: ....

Sleep	Weight	Blood Pressure	Fluids Intake

Feeling: ....

DRUGS & MEDICATIONS	DOSAGE	TIMING

MEALS	TIME	NOTES

Tasks & Activities

....

....

....

....

Concerns / Notes

....

....

....

Daily Journal

Date:
....

Caregiver:
....

Sleep	Weight	Blood Pressure	Fluids Intake

Fluids Intake symbols: ▢ ▢ ▢ ▢ ▢ ▢ ▢ ▢

Feeling:
....

DRUGS & MEDICATIONS	DOSAGE	TIMING

MEALS	TIME	NOTES

Tasks & Activities

....

....

....

....

Concerns / Notes

....

....

....

....

Daily Journal

Date:

Caregiver:

Sleep	Weight	Blood Pressure	Fluids Intake

Feeling:

DRUGS & MEDICATIONS	DOSAGE	TIMING

MEALS	TIME	NOTES

Tasks & Activities

Concerns / Notes

Daily Journal

Date: ....

Caregiver: ....

Sleep	Weight	Blood Pressure	Fluids Intake

Feeling: ....

DRUGS & MEDICATIONS	DOSAGE	TIMING

MEALS	TIME	NOTES

Tasks & Activities

....

....

....

....

Concerns / Notes

....

....

....

....

Daily Journal

Date:

Caregiver:

Sleep	Weight	Blood Pressure	Fluids Intake

Feeling:

DRUGS & MEDICATIONS	DOSAGE	TIMING

MEALS	TIME	NOTES

Tasks & Activities

Concerns / Notes

Daily Journal

Date:
....

Caregiver:
....

Sleep	Weight	Blood Pressure	Fluids Intake

Feeling:
....

DRUGS & MEDICATIONS	DOSAGE	TIMING

MEALS	TIME	NOTES

Tasks & Activities
....
....
....
....

Concerns / Notes
....
....
....
....

Daily Journal

Caregiver:

Date:

Sleep	Weight	Blood Pressure	Fluids Intake

Feeling:

DRUGS & MEDICATIONS	DOSAGE	TIMING

MEALS	TIME	NOTES

Tasks & Activities

Concerns / Notes

Daily Journal

Date:

Caregiver:

Sleep	Weight	Blood Pressure	Fluids Intake

Feeling:

DRUGS & MEDICATIONS	DOSAGE	TIMING

MEALS	TIME	NOTES

Tasks & Activities

Concerns / Notes

Daily Journal

Date:

Caregiver:

Sleep	Weight	Blood Pressure	Fluids Intake

Feeling:

DRUGS & MEDICATIONS	DOSAGE	TIMING

MEALS	TIME	NOTES

Tasks & Activities

Concerns / Notes

Daily Journal

Date:

Caregiver:

Sleep	Weight	Blood Pressure	Fluids Intake

Feeling:

DRUGS & MEDICATIONS	DOSAGE	TIMING

MEALS	TIME	NOTES

Tasks & Activities

Concerns / Notes

Daily Journal

Date:

Caregiver:

Sleep	Weight	Blood Pressure	Fluids Intake

Feeling:

DRUGS & MEDICATIONS	DOSAGE	TIMING

MEALS	TIME	NOTES

Tasks & Activities

Concerns / Notes

Daily Journal

Date: ....

Caregiver: ....

Sleep	Weight	Blood Pressure	Fluids Intake

Feeling: ....

DRUGS & MEDICATIONS	DOSAGE	TIMING

MEALS	TIME	NOTES

Tasks & Activities

....

....

....

....

Concerns / Notes

....

....

....

....

Daily Journal

Date: ....

Caregiver: ....

Sleep	Weight	Blood Pressure	Fluids Intake

Feeling: ....

DRUGS & MEDICATIONS	DOSAGE	TIMING

MEALS	TIME	NOTES

Tasks & Activities

....

....

....

....

Concerns / Notes

....

....

....

Daily Journal

Date:
....

Caregiver:
....

Sleep	Weight	Blood Pressure	Fluids Intake

Feeling:
....

DRUGS & MEDICATIONS		DOSAGE	TIMING

MEALS	TIME		NOTES

Tasks & Activities
....
....
....
....

Concerns / Notes
....
....
....
....
....

Daily Journal

Date: ....

Caregiver: ....

Sleep	Weight	Blood Pressure	Fluids Intake

Feeling: ....

DRUGS & MEDICATIONS	DOSAGE	TIMING

MEALS	TIME	NOTES

Tasks & Activities

....

....

....

....

Concerns / Notes

....

....

....

....

Daily Journal

Date: ....

Caregiver: ....

Sleep	Weight	Blood Pressure	Fluids Intake

Feeling: ....

DRUGS & MEDICATIONS	DOSAGE	TIMING

MEALS	TIME	NOTES

Tasks & Activities

....

....

....

....

Concerns / Notes

....

....

....

....

Daily Journal

Date: ....

Caregiver: ....

Sleep	Weight	Blood Pressure	Fluids Intake

Feeling: ....

DRUGS & MEDICATIONS	DOSAGE	TIMING

MEALS	TIME	NOTES

Tasks & Activities

....

....

....

....

Concerns / Notes

....

....

....

Daily Journal

Date: ....

Caregiver: ....

Sleep	Weight	Blood Pressure	Fluids Intake

Feeling: ....

DRUGS & MEDICATIONS	DOSAGE	TIMING

MEALS	TIME	NOTES

Tasks & Activities

....

....

....

....

Concerns / Notes

....

....

....

....

....

Daily Journal

Date: ....

Caregiver: ....

Sleep	Weight	Blood Pressure	Fluids Intake

Feeling: ....

DRUGS & MEDICATIONS	DOSAGE	TIMING

MEALS	TIME	NOTES

Tasks & Activities

....

....

....

....

Concerns / Notes

....

....

....

....

Daily Journal

Date: ....

Caregiver: ....

Sleep	Weight	Blood Pressure	Fluids Intake

Feeling: ....

DRUGS & MEDICATIONS	DOSAGE	TIMING

MEALS	TIME	NOTES

Tasks & Activities

....
....
....
....

Concerns / Notes

....
....
....
....

Daily Journal

Date: ....

Caregiver: ....

Sleep	Weight	Blood Pressure	Fluids Intake

Feeling: ....

DRUGS & MEDICATIONS	DOSAGE	TIMING

MEALS	TIME	NOTES

Tasks & Activities

....

....

....

....

Concerns / Notes

....

....

....

....

Daily Journal

Date: ....

Caregiver: ....

Sleep	Weight	Blood Pressure	Fluids Intake

Feeling: ....

DRUGS & MEDICATIONS	DOSAGE	TIMING

MEALS	TIME	NOTES

Tasks & Activities

....

....

....

....

Concerns / Notes

....

....

....

....

Daily Journal

Date: ....

Caregiver: ....

Sleep	Weight	Blood Pressure	Fluids Intake

Feeling: ....

DRUGS & MEDICATIONS	DOSAGE	TIMING

MEALS	TIME	NOTES

Tasks & Activities

....

....

....

....

Concerns / Notes

....

....

....

....

Daily Journal

Date:
....

Caregiver:
....

Sleep	Weight	Blood Pressure	Fluids Intake

Feeling:
....

DRUGS & MEDICATIONS	DOSAGE	TIMING

MEALS	TIME	NOTES

Tasks & Activities

....

....

....

....

Concerns / Notes

....

....

....

....

Daily Journal

Date: ....

Caregiver: ....

Sleep	Weight	Blood Pressure	Fluids Intake

Feeling: ....

DRUGS & MEDICATIONS	DOSAGE	TIMING

MEALS	TIME	NOTES

Tasks & Activities

....

....

....

....

Concerns / Notes

....

....

....

....

Daily Journal

Date:

Caregiver:

Sleep	Weight	Blood Pressure	Fluids Intake

Feeling:

DRUGS & MEDICATIONS	DOSAGE	TIMING

MEALS	TIME	NOTES

Tasks & Activities

Concerns / Notes

Daily Journal

Date: ....

Caregiver: ....

Sleep	Weight	Blood Pressure	Fluids Intake

Feeling: ....

DRUGS & MEDICATIONS	DOSAGE	TIMING

MEALS	TIME	NOTES

Tasks & Activities

....

....

....

Concerns / Notes

....

....

....

....

Daily Journal

Date:

Caregiver:

Sleep	Weight	Blood Pressure	Fluids Intake

Feeling:

DRUGS & MEDICATIONS	DOSAGE	TIMING

MEALS	TIME	NOTES

Tasks & Activities

Concerns / Notes

Daily Journal

Date: ....

Caregiver: ....

Sleep	Weight	Blood Pressure	Fluids Intake

Feeling: ....

DRUGS & MEDICATIONS	DOSAGE	TIMING

MEALS	TIME	NOTES

Tasks & Activities

....

....

....

....

Concerns / Notes

....

....

....

Daily Journal

Date: ....

Caregiver: ....

Sleep	Weight	Blood Pressure	Fluids Intake

Feeling: ....

DRUGS & MEDICATIONS	DOSAGE	TIMING

MEALS	TIME	NOTES

Tasks & Activities

....

....

....

....

Concerns / Notes

....

....

....

....

Daily Journal

Date: ....

Caregiver: ....

Sleep	Weight	Blood Pressure	Fluids Intake

Feeling: ....

DRUGS & MEDICATIONS	DOSAGE	TIMING

MEALS	TIME	NOTES

Tasks & Activities

....

....

....

....

Concerns / Notes

....

....

....

....

Daily Journal

Date:

Caregiver:

Sleep	Weight	Blood Pressure	Fluids Intake

Feeling:

DRUGS & MEDICATIONS	DOSAGE	TIMING

MEALS	TIME	NOTES

Tasks & Activities

Concerns / Notes

Daily Journal

Date:

Caregiver:

Sleep	Weight	Blood Pressure	Fluids Intake

Feeling:

DRUGS & MEDICATIONS	DOSAGE	TIMING

MEALS	TIME	NOTES

Tasks & Activities

Concerns / Notes

Daily Journal

Date: ....

Caregiver: ....

Sleep	Weight	Blood Pressure	Fluids Intake

Feeling: ....

DRUGS & MEDICATIONS	DOSAGE	TIMING

MEALS	TIME	NOTES

Tasks & Activities
....
....
....
....

Concerns / Notes
....
....
....
....
....

Daily Journal

Date:

Caregiver:

Sleep	Weight	Blood Pressure	Fluids Intake

Feeling:

DRUGS & MEDICATIONS	DOSAGE	TIMING

MEALS	TIME	NOTES

Tasks & Activities

Concerns / Notes

Daily Journal

Date: ....

Caregiver: ....

Sleep	Weight	Blood Pressure	Fluids Intake

Feeling: ....

DRUGS & MEDICATIONS	DOSAGE	TIMING

MEALS	TIME	NOTES

Tasks & Activities

....

....

....

....

Concerns / Notes

....

....

....

Daily Journal

Date:

Caregiver:

Sleep	Weight	Blood Pressure	Fluids Intake

Feeling:

DRUGS & MEDICATIONS		DOSAGE	TIMING

MEALS	TIME	NOTES

Tasks & Activities

Concerns / Notes

Daily Journal

Date:

Caregiver:

Sleep	Weight	Blood Pressure	Fluids Intake

Feeling:

DRUGS & MEDICATIONS	DOSAGE	TIMING

MEALS	TIME	NOTES

Tasks & Activities

Concerns / Notes

Daily Journal

Date:

Caregiver:

Sleep	Weight	Blood Pressure	Fluids Intake

Feeling:

DRUGS & MEDICATIONS	DOSAGE	TIMING

MEALS	TIME	NOTES

Tasks & Activities

Concerns / Notes

Daily Journal

Date: ....

Caregiver: ....

Sleep	Weight	Blood Pressure	Fluids Intake

Fluids Intake: ⊔ ⊔ ⊔ ⊔ ⊔ ⊔ ⊔ ⊔

Feeling: ....

DRUGS & MEDICATIONS	DOSAGE	TIMING

MEALS	TIME	NOTES

Tasks & Activities

....

....

....

....

Concerns / Notes

....

....

....

....

Daily Journal

Date:

Caregiver:

Sleep	Weight	Blood Pressure	Fluids Intake

Feeling:

DRUGS & MEDICATIONS	DOSAGE	TIMING

MEALS	TIME	NOTES

Tasks & Activities

Concerns / Notes

Daily Journal

Date:

Caregiver:

Sleep	Weight	Blood Pressure	Fluids Intake

Feeling:

DRUGS & MEDICATIONS	DOSAGE	TIMING

MEALS	TIME	NOTES

Tasks & Activities

Concerns / Notes

Daily Journal

Date:

Caregiver:

Sleep	Weight	Blood Pressure	Fluids Intake

Feeling:

DRUGS & MEDICATIONS		DOSAGE	TIMING

MEALS	TIME		NOTES

Tasks & Activities

Concerns / Notes

Daily Journal

Date:
....

Caregiver:
....

Sleep	Weight	Blood Pressure	Fluids Intake

Feeling:
....

DRUGS & MEDICATIONS	DOSAGE	TIMING

MEALS	TIME	NOTES

Tasks & Activities
....
....
....
....

Concerns / Notes
....
....
....
....

Daily Journal

Date: ....

Caregiver: ....

Sleep	Weight	Blood Pressure	Fluids Intake

Feeling: ....

DRUGS & MEDICATIONS	DOSAGE	TIMING

MEALS	TIME	NOTES

Tasks & Activities

....

....

....

Concerns / Notes

....

....

....

Daily Journal

Date:
....

Caregiver:
....

Sleep	Weight	Blood Pressure	Fluids Intake

Feeling:
....

DRUGS & MEDICATIONS	DOSAGE	TIMING

MEALS	TIME	NOTES

Tasks & Activities
....
....
....
....

Concerns / Notes
....
....
....
....

Daily Journal

Date: ....

Caregiver: ....

Sleep	Weight	Blood Pressure	Fluids Intake

Feeling: ....

DRUGS & MEDICATIONS	DOSAGE	TIMING

MEALS	TIME	NOTES

Tasks & Activities

....

....

....

....

Concerns / Notes

....

....

....

....

Daily Journal

Date: ....

Caregiver: ....

Sleep	Weight	Blood Pressure	Fluids Intake

Feeling: ....

DRUGS & MEDICATIONS	DOSAGE	TIMING

MEALS	TIME	NOTES

Tasks & Activities

....

....

....

....

Concerns / Notes

....

....

....

....

Daily Journal

Date:

Caregiver:

Sleep	Weight	Blood Pressure	Fluids Intake

Feeling:

DRUGS & MEDICATIONS	DOSAGE	TIMING

MEALS	TIME	NOTES

Tasks & Activities

Concerns / Notes

Daily Journal

Date:

Caregiver:

Sleep	Weight	Blood Pressure	Fluids Intake

Feeling:

DRUGS & MEDICATIONS	DOSAGE	TIMING

MEALS	TIME	NOTES

Tasks & Activities

Concerns / Notes

Daily Journal

Date: ....

Caregiver: ....

Sleep	Weight	Blood Pressure	Fluids Intake

Feeling: ....

DRUGS & MEDICATIONS	DOSAGE	TIMING

MEALS	TIME	NOTES

Tasks & Activities

....
....
....
....

Concerns / Notes

....
....
....
....

Daily Journal

Date:

Caregiver:

Sleep	Weight	Blood Pressure	Fluids Intake

Feeling:

DRUGS & MEDICATIONS	DOSAGE	TIMING

MEALS	TIME	NOTES

Tasks & Activities

Concerns / Notes

Daily Journal

Date:

Caregiver:

Sleep	Weight	Blood Pressure	Fluids Intake
			⊔⊔⊔⊔⊔⊔⊔⊔

Feeling:

DRUGS & MEDICATIONS	DOSAGE	TIMING

MEALS	TIME	NOTES

Tasks & Activities

Concerns / Notes

Daily Journal

Date: ....

Caregiver: ....

Sleep	Weight	Blood Pressure	Fluids Intake

Feeling: ....

DRUGS & MEDICATIONS	DOSAGE	TIMING

MEALS	TIME	NOTES

Tasks & Activities
....
....
....
....

Concerns / Notes
....
....
....
....
....

Daily Journal

Date:

Caregiver:

Sleep	Weight	Blood Pressure	Fluids Intake

Feeling:

DRUGS & MEDICATIONS	DOSAGE	TIMING

MEALS	TIME	NOTES

Tasks & Activities

Concerns / Notes

Daily Journal

Date: ....

Caregiver: ....

Sleep	Weight	Blood Pressure	Fluids Intake

Feeling: ....

DRUGS & MEDICATIONS	DOSAGE	TIMING

MEALS	TIME	NOTES

Tasks & Activities

....

....

....

Concerns / Notes

....

....

....

....

Daily Journal

Date: ....

Caregiver: ....

Sleep	Weight	Blood Pressure	Fluids Intake

Feeling: ....

DRUGS & MEDICATIONS	DOSAGE	TIMING

MEALS	TIME	NOTES

Tasks & Activities

....

....

....

....

Concerns / Notes

....

....

....

....

Daily Journal

Date:

Caregiver:

Sleep	Weight	Blood Pressure	Fluids Intake

Feeling:

DRUGS & MEDICATIONS	DOSAGE	TIMING

MEALS	TIME	NOTES

Tasks & Activities

Concerns / Notes

Daily Journal

Date:

Caregiver:

Sleep	Weight	Blood Pressure	Fluids Intake

Feeling:

DRUGS & MEDICATIONS	DOSAGE	TIMING

MEALS	TIME	NOTES

Tasks & Activities

Concerns / Notes

Daily Journal

Date: ....

Caregiver: ....

Sleep	Weight	Blood Pressure	Fluids Intake

Feeling: ....

DRUGS & MEDICATIONS	DOSAGE	TIMING

MEALS	TIME	NOTES

Tasks & Activities

....

....

....

....

Concerns / Notes

....

....

....

....

Daily Journal

Date: ....

Caregiver: ....

Sleep	Weight	Blood Pressure	Fluids Intake

Feeling: ....

DRUGS & MEDICATIONS	DOSAGE	TIMING

MEALS	TIME	NOTES

Tasks & Activities

Concerns / Notes

Daily Journal

Date:

Caregiver:

Sleep	Weight	Blood Pressure	Fluids Intake

Feeling:

DRUGS & MEDICATIONS	DOSAGE	TIMING

MEALS	TIME	NOTES

Tasks & Activities

Concerns / Notes

Daily Journal

Date:

Caregiver:

Sleep	Weight	Blood Pressure	Fluids Intake

Feeling:

DRUGS & MEDICATIONS	DOSAGE	TIMING

MEALS	TIME	NOTES

Tasks & Activities

Concerns / Notes

Daily Journal

Date: ....

Caregiver: ....

Sleep	Weight	Blood Pressure	Fluids Intake

Feeling: ....

DRUGS & MEDICATIONS	DOSAGE	TIMING

MEALS	TIME	NOTES

Tasks & Activities

....

....

....

....

Concerns / Notes

....

....

....

....

Daily Journal

Date:

Caregiver:

Sleep	Weight	Blood Pressure	Fluids Intake

Feeling:

DRUGS & MEDICATIONS	DOSAGE	TIMING

MEALS	TIME	NOTES

Tasks & Activities

Concerns / Notes

Daily Journal

Date:

Caregiver:

Sleep	Weight	Blood Pressure	Fluids Intake

Feeling:

DRUGS & MEDICATIONS	DOSAGE	TIMING

MEALS	TIME	NOTES

Tasks & Activities

Concerns / Notes

Daily Journal

Date:

Caregiver:

Sleep	Weight	Blood Pressure	Fluids Intake

Feeling:

DRUGS & MEDICATIONS	DOSAGE	TIMING

MEALS	TIME	NOTES

Tasks & Activities

Concerns / Notes

Daily Journal

Date: ....

Caregiver: ....

Sleep	Weight	Blood Pressure	Fluids Intake

Feeling: ....

DRUGS & MEDICATIONS	DOSAGE	TIMING

MEALS	TIME	NOTES

Tasks & Activities

....

....

....

....

Concerns / Notes

....

....

....

....

Daily Journal

Date:

Caregiver:

Sleep	Weight	Blood Pressure	Fluids Intake

Feeling:

DRUGS & MEDICATIONS	DOSAGE	TIMING

MEALS	TIME	NOTES

Tasks & Activities

Concerns / Notes

Daily Journal

Date:
....

Caregiver:
....

Sleep	Weight	Blood Pressure	Fluids Intake

Feeling:
....

DRUGS & MEDICATIONS	DOSAGE	TIMING

MEALS	TIME	NOTES

Tasks & Activities
....
....
....
....

Concerns / Notes
....
....
....
....

Daily Journal

Date:

Caregiver:

Sleep	Weight	Blood Pressure	Fluids Intake

Feeling:

DRUGS & MEDICATIONS	DOSAGE	TIMING

MEALS	TIME	NOTES

Tasks & Activities

Concerns / Notes

Daily Journal

Date:

Caregiver:

Sleep	Weight	Blood Pressure	Fluids Intake

Feeling:

DRUGS & MEDICATIONS	DOSAGE	TIMING

MEALS	TIME	NOTES

Tasks & Activities

Concerns / Notes

Daily Journal

Date:

Caregiver:

Sleep	Weight	Blood Pressure	Fluids Intake

Feeling:

DRUGS & MEDICATIONS	DOSAGE	TIMING

MEALS	TIME	NOTES

Tasks & Activities

Concerns / Notes

Daily Journal

Date: ....

Caregiver: ....

Sleep	Weight	Blood Pressure	Fluids Intake

Feeling: ....

DRUGS & MEDICATIONS	DOSAGE	TIMING

MEALS	TIME	NOTES

Tasks & Activities

....

....

....

....

Concerns / Notes

....

....

....

....

Daily Journal

Date:

Caregiver:

Sleep	Weight	Blood Pressure	Fluids Intake

Feeling:

DRUGS & MEDICATIONS	DOSAGE	TIMING

MEALS	TIME	NOTES

Tasks & Activities

Concerns / Notes

Daily Journal

Caregiver: ....

Date: ....

Sleep	Weight	Blood Pressure	Fluids Intake

Feeling: ....

DRUGS & MEDICATIONS	DOSAGE	TIMING

MEALS	TIME	NOTES

Tasks & Activities

....

....

....

....

Concerns / Notes

....

....

....

....

Daily Journal

Date: ....

Caregiver: ....

Sleep	Weight	Blood Pressure	Fluids Intake

Fluids Intake ⊔ ⊔ ⊔ ⊔ ⊔ ⊔ ⊔ ⊔

Feeling: ....

DRUGS & MEDICATIONS	DOSAGE	TIMING

MEALS	TIME	NOTES

Tasks & Activities

....

....

....

....

Concerns / Notes

....

....

....

....

Daily Journal

Caregiver:

Date:

Sleep	Weight	Blood Pressure	Fluids Intake

Feeling:

DRUGS & MEDICATIONS	DOSAGE	TIMING

MEALS	TIME	NOTES

Tasks & Activities

Concerns / Notes

Daily Journal

Date:

Caregiver:

Sleep	Weight	Blood Pressure	Fluids Intake

Feeling:

DRUGS & MEDICATIONS	DOSAGE	TIMING

MEALS	TIME	NOTES

Tasks & Activities

Concerns / Notes

Daily Journal

Date: ....

Caregiver: ....

Sleep	Weight	Blood Pressure	Fluids Intake

Feeling: ....

DRUGS & MEDICATIONS	DOSAGE	TIMING

MEALS	TIME	NOTES

Tasks & Activities

....

....

....

....

Concerns / Notes

....

....

....

....

Daily Journal

Date:

Caregiver:

Sleep	Weight	Blood Pressure	Fluids Intake

Feeling:

DRUGS & MEDICATIONS	DOSAGE	TIMING

MEALS	TIME	NOTES

Tasks & Activities

Concerns / Notes

Daily Journal

Caregiver: ....

Date: ....

Sleep	Weight	Blood Pressure	Fluids Intake

Feeling: ....

DRUGS & MEDICATIONS	DOSAGE	TIMING

MEALS	TIME	NOTES

Tasks & Activities

....

....

....

....

Concerns / Notes

....

....

....

....

Daily Journal

Caregiver:

Date:

Sleep	Weight	Blood Pressure	Fluids Intake

Feeling:

DRUGS & MEDICATIONS	DOSAGE	TIMING

MEALS	TIME	NOTES

Tasks & Activities

Concerns / Notes

Daily Journal

Date:

Caregiver:

Sleep	Weight	Blood Pressure	Fluids Intake

Feeling:

DRUGS & MEDICATIONS	DOSAGE	TIMING

MEALS	TIME	NOTES

Tasks & Activities

Concerns / Notes

Daily Journal

Date:

Caregiver:

Sleep	Weight	Blood Pressure	Fluids Intake

Feeling:

DRUGS & MEDICATIONS	DOSAGE	TIMING

MEALS	TIME	NOTES

Tasks & Activities

Concerns / Notes

Daily Journal

Date: ....

Caregiver: ....

Sleep	Weight	Blood Pressure	Fluids Intake

Feeling: ....

DRUGS & MEDICATIONS	DOSAGE	TIMING

MEALS	TIME	NOTES

Tasks & Activities

....

....

....

....

Concerns / Notes

....

....

....

....

Daily Journal

Caregiver: ....

Date: ....

Sleep	Weight	Blood Pressure	Fluids Intake

Feeling: ....

DRUGS & MEDICATIONS	DOSAGE	TIMING

MEALS	TIME	NOTES

Tasks & Activities

....

....

....

....

Concerns / Notes

....

....

....

....

Daily Journal

Date: ....

Caregiver: ....

Sleep	Weight	Blood Pressure	Fluids Intake

Feeling: ....

DRUGS & MEDICATIONS	DOSAGE	TIMING

MEALS	TIME	NOTES

Tasks & Activities

....

....

....

....

Concerns / Notes

....

....

....

....

Daily Journal

Date:

Caregiver:

Sleep	Weight	Blood Pressure	Fluids Intake								

Feeling:

DRUGS & MEDICATIONS	DOSAGE	TIMING

MEALS	TIME	NOTES

Tasks & Activities

Concerns / Notes

Daily Journal

Date:

Caregiver:

Sleep	Weight	Blood Pressure	Fluids Intake

Feeling:

DRUGS & MEDICATIONS	DOSAGE	TIMING

MEALS	TIME	NOTES

Tasks & Activities

Concerns / Notes

Daily Journal

Caregiver:

Sleep	Weight	Blood Pressure	Fluids Intake

Feeling:

DRUGS & MEDICATIONS	DOSAGE	TIMING

MEALS	TIME	NOTES	

Tasks & Activities

Concerns / Notes

Daily Journal

Date: ....

Caregiver: ....

Sleep	Weight	Blood Pressure	Fluids Intake

Feeling: ....

DRUGS & MEDICATIONS	DOSAGE	TIMING

MEALS	TIME	NOTES

Tasks & Activities

....

....

....

....

Concerns / Notes

....

....

....

....

Daily Journal

Date: ....

Caregiver: ....

Sleep	Weight	Blood Pressure	Fluids Intake

Feeling: ....

DRUGS & MEDICATIONS	DOSAGE	TIMING

MEALS	TIME	NOTES

Tasks & Activities

....

....

....

Concerns / Notes

....

....

....

Month:

Sunday	Monday	Tuesday	Wednesday	Thursday	Friday	Saturday
Notes:						

Month:

Sunday	Monday	Tuesday	Wednesday	Thursday	Friday	Saturday
☐	☐	☐	☐	☐	☐	☐
☐	☐	☐	☐	☐	☐	☐
☐	☐	☐	☐	☐	☐	☐
☐	☐	☐	☐	☐	☐	☐
☐	☐	☐	☐	☐	☐	☐
☐	☐	Notes:				

Month:

Sunday	Monday	Tuesday	Wednesday	Thursday	Friday	Saturday
☐	☐	☐	☐	☐	☐	☐
☐	☐	☐	☐	☐	☐	☐
☐	☐	☐	☐	☐	☐	☐
☐	☐	☐	☐	☐	☐	☐
☐	☐	☐	☐	☐	☐	☐
☐	☐	Notes:				

Month:

Sunday	Monday	Tuesday	Wednesday	Thursday	Friday	Saturday
☐	☐	☐	☐	☐	☐	☐
☐	☐	☐	☐	☐	☐	☐
☐	☐	☐	☐	☐	☐	☐
☐	☐	☐	☐	☐	☐	☐
☐	☐	☐	☐	☐	☐	☐
☐	☐	Notes:				

Notes

Notes

Notes